"Why Do I Still Hurt?"

Rapid Relief for Chronic Pain, Depression, Anxiety, and More!

Discover the **Hidden Causes** Behind Your Pain & Suffering, and a Revolutionary Healing Method for Release & Relief… Starting NOW!

BY
DEBORA WAYNE

DEDICATION PAGE

Thirty-one years ago, at the very instant when I thought the pain in all areas of my life could not possibly get any worse, I experienced a "divine moment," and I became open. Open - and teachable - for the first time in years ... perhaps for the first time ever.

It was at that critical crossroads moment that a very wise woman, a true angel in human form, appeared in the movie of my life and spoke these wise words to me:

"Deb, The truth, is the shortcut. Tell the truth and go **through** *each experience, not around, to gain the gift of true freedom from pain and suffering."*

It is with profound gratitude that I dedicate this book to Angie, my "messenger," who raised me up from the dead and returned me to the land of the living. I am, and will remain, eternally grateful.

FOREWORD

Pain.
It's everywhere.

No matter where I am, I notice indications of people suffering from some type of pain and/or dis-ease.

I see it in their faces. I hear it in their voices. I feel it when I'm with them.

The checkout line at every grocery store contains glaring reminders that we must prepare for inevitable pain and sickness. Remedies for headaches, winter colds, flu, acid indigestion, sleep deprivation, jet lag, low energy, and more, compete for center stage. These have become as common and necessary as food - a staple of modern life.

Almost every television ad offers yet another drug for those suffering from disease, depression, aches, anxiety, and pain.

The reminders of the inevitability of pain and dis-ease are everywhere!

It begs the question: Why are we all in such pain ... and more importantly, *how do we find true relief?*

As a pain release and energy expert, I've worked with thousands and thousands of people from all around the world. Although they all experience different symptoms, each one of them, without fail, has said to me: "Debora, "Why do I still hurt? I've tried **everything** to get rid of my pain and symptoms, but nothing seems to help, or if it does, the results don't last."

This question, *"Why Do I Still Hurt?"* has haunted me, kept me awake many nights, nagged at me, appeared and reappeared, until I answered it's call.

I've immersed myself in this subject day and night for many years, and now I hope you'll join me on this journey.

This book is designed to begin what I believe is an important—and often completely overlooked—conversation.

I hope to wake you up, and shake you up, and entice you to look deeper—below the surface of your painful symptoms. When you do, I'm confident you'll gain a new understanding, an unconventional perspective, on the often overlooked, underlying root cause of all pain and suffering.

Now, this root cause is rarely spoken about, and most likely will not be indicated on medical tests ... even when using the most sophisticated technology or equipment.

In fact, this root cause of pain is embedded in your history and your unconscious mind, even though you are likely not aware of it just yet.

Most importantly, I want to share with you information about a revolutionary, scientifically proven, yet unfamiliar, healing method that has helped thousands of my past clients in over 150 countries to completely eliminate their Chronic Pain, Depression, Anxiety, Trauma, Immune weakness, Digestive Disorders, Binge-Eating, Weight issues, and much much more, without the use of any drugs, supplements, surgeries, or lengthy or invasive treatments.

It's time to open your eyes now to new possibilities.

Relief *is* possible, and it may be easier than you think.

> *"Sometimes I've believed as many as six impossible things before breakfast."*
> --- Lewis Carroll

It would be an impossible task to cover everything I'd like to share with you in this book ... everything I've learned from over 30+ years of my personal and professional health and healing journey. **So if while you read, you find the material really resonating with you, or perhaps you already know that you are ready right now to dive in and receive my personal help... Then simply join me here: www.BiofieldHealingInstitute.com/dohps**

Before You Begin
Before we get started, I'd like to make sure you have everything you need to get the absolute most out of this experience.

Follow the steps below to prepare.

Then, buckle your seat belt and open yourself to a brand new experience! I understand, from your current perspective, from where you are right now, you probably do not realize what's possible for you ... but I promise you, thousands of my past clients have reported complete and total healing from serious, chronic pain and dis-ease even though they had tried everything and were told 'this will never change'. Now, I'd like to add *you* to that list!

Step 1.
Grab some paper and something to write with. In addition to taking notes on the sections of this book that resonate most with you, we're going to go through

s .

some exercises that require you to write down your thoughts and insights, so this journey is both personal and meaningful, and perhaps even life-changing, for you! Carry this pen and paper around with you! Keep it next to your bed … write down your thoughts, feelings, and dreams as they come up.

Make it a new habit to notice what you're thinking and how you're feeling. This is the first step toward healing.

Step 2.
Commit to being fully present. As you read, limit your distractions. Commit to being here fully, commit to yourself, and open up to a new experience. This will ensure you gain the healing and transformation this book is meant to facilitate. Turn off your email, your phone, and your social media accounts.
Give yourself 100% focus, attention, and intention.

Step 3.
Be willing. Open yourself up to finally being willing to see what's really stopping and blocking you, and getting in your way. Ask yourself the questions I ask you to consider as you read, and let the answers come to you. Your answers ARE there. The first answers that come up are often the most accurate. Trust this process.
Be willing and open to receiving your answers: this simple and very important act will allow you to receive the greatest benefits.

Step 4.
Set aside your worries! If you're worried that you're too blocked or too stuck, or in too much pain to receive healing, that's simply not the case. The solution may seem hidden from your view at the moment, but I want to remind you that *anything* is possible. Your willingness is key. Trust the process. Different people grow at different rates, so never compare your results to others. *The more you can let go and trust this process, the better results you'll experience!*
Often, the answers come when you least expect them.

Step 5.
Say, "Yes!" Decide, right now, that you're going to let the healing begin!

Please note: If as you read this book you begin to experience any of the following: head pressure, nausea, drowsiness, difficulty paying attention, yawning, feeling "spacey", or other symptoms, please know this is just your body responding perfectly to the healing frequencies you need which are being transmitted to you (yes, even through a book)! Do your best not to worry or resist this and certainly don't fight it. Typically it will integrate and the symptoms should pass very quickly. You'll understand more about this

as you read, so for now please just trust the process and know that, when your body reacts, you **ARE** receiving healing.

Now, are you ready?

Let's get started!

"This body Arjuna, is called the field.
He who knows this is called the knower of the field."
—*Bhagavad Gita 13:1*

INTRODUCTION

Welcome!
You are here for an important reason although you may not understand "the why" yet at all.

I've learned and experienced so much in this amazing lifetime, and I've come to understand that *there are no accidents.*

If any of the following sound familiar, you ARE in the right place, and most importantly, *there is hope.*

- You've experienced pain, illness, anxiety or depression for so long now that *you almost don't remember what it feels like to feel good.* You have stopped dreaming, and have begun to feel hopeless, like there is no solution for what ails you.
- *You've tried so many different healing modalities,* you could write a book on them … but none of them have worked well for long periods of time.
- You want to heal at a deeper level, *so you don't have to rely on drugs to mask your symptoms.*
- Doctors have told you to "just live with it," but *you're just not ready to give up.*
- You're frustrated, discouraged and *afraid there is nothing out there to help you.*

Or …

- You're a healthcare practitioner and *you are looking for new ways to help your clients go beyond the limitations of the current methods you practice, to bring them relief and healing.*

Trust me, I hear it ALL the time - you feel like you've tried everything: nutrition, psychiatry, anti-depressants, anti-anxiety medications, medical marijuana, opioids, surgery, supplements, physical therapy, yoga, chiropractors, Rolfing, personal training, religion, acupuncture, elimination diets, anti-inflammatory diets, food plans, exercise, fasting, cleanses, juicing,, meditation, massage therapy, and more … but you've achieved little, partial, or even *zero* results. Nada. Null.

Now, you're angry, discouraged, and frustrated. It's so hard to live in pain all the time, and you want out!

Sound familiar?

If so, I want you to take a deep, cleansing breath, right now. (Really – relax your low belly and inhale through your nose for a count of 5, and exhale through your mouth for the same. Repeat a few times, until you feel the calm come over you.)

If you've lost hope, please don't. What you'll discover in this book is possible for *you*, too!

The field of health is changing, dramatically. In fact, there's a health and healing revolution going on, right now, and you are part of it, whether you realize it or not.

You're about to discover a completely different approach to your own health and well-being - one that is based in science, and rooted in research, and also deeply connected to ancient spiritual traditions.

Before I dive in, though, I want you to consider this: at one time, people believed the earth was flat. Not just one or two people … this was a widely held belief *most* people considered truth. Obviously, we all know now that the earth is round.

I'm asking *you* now to open your mind, to what may seem like new and unfamiliar truths.

Please keep an open mind as you read. You may be shocked by what is possible for you.

I'll explain why poor health is *not* inevitable as you age … why *all illness has the potential to change… and why your focus on "what's wrong" may actually be killing you.*

Please suspend (even just temporarily) any doubts you may have. I know it can feel frightening to leave what's familiar, even if what's familiar is harming you – but I encourage you to do exactly that – free yourself from the confines of beliefs that may not be serving you, and explore seeing from a new perspective, starting right now.

***

Pain, illness, and stress have become chronic problems for so many people in today's fast-paced world.

Everyone seems to be in some kind of pain, whether it's physical, like back pain, stomach aches, arthritis, hip and shoulder pain, or emotional, such as low self-esteem, lack of confidence, anxiety, depression, guilt, or grief.

People often suffer from feeling a lack of love, hating their careers, and/or feeling out of control of their finances, too.

Dis-ease shows its face in so many facets, all over the world.

- It is estimated that approximately **1 out of 6 Americans**, some 50 million people, **experience the wrath of chronic pain** (3 months or more of pain) during the course of a year.
- The American Academy of Pain Medicine reports that **chronic pain affects more Americans than heart disease, diabetes and cancer combined.**

- Employees suffering from chronic pain **miss more than 50 million days of work annually.**
- According to a survey by The American Psychological Association (APA), **two-thirds of Americans said they were likely to seek help for the effects of stress.**
- **73% of Americans name money as their number one stress factor** (and stress is always the pre-curser to pain and dis-ease..
- Harvard Medical School found that **people with chronic pain are three times more likely to develop symptoms of depression.**

That being said, have you ever wondered why some people seem to heal quickly from pain or illness, while others experience little to no results at all?

Why do some people go through life filled with energy and vitality, while others are chronically fatigued, sick, or injured?

Most importantly, how is it that, in this sophisticated, 21st-Century information-rich age, people often can't get the relief they so badly want and need?

The answer is simple: When we look only to the physical body for answers, we're looking in the wrong place.

To truly understand this answer, we'll have to examine a different take on health, and delve into some complex ideas. (This is where keeping that open mind comes in!)

You see, under our current medical model, doctors and other health professionals treat *symptoms*. We are focused on symptoms, on disease ... *not* on health.

In our culture, we have been conditioned to believe that taking medication to suppress symptoms equates to healing.

But, symptoms are not the root cause. Focusing on symptoms is like watering the leaves of a tree hoping it will keep the tree healthy. It won't happen!

When you don't know and aren't treating the root cause, you don't experience actual healing.

Yet the current medical model typically focuses solely on the body - but there is so much more to your health than that.

YOU are not your body.

You *have* a body, and your body shares an intricate and inseparable connection with your mind and your emotions.

Just like everything else in this universe, you are made up of vibrating particles of energy. Energy never dies, yet it can (and does) change form all the time.

I like to explain this using an ice cube analogy.

An ice cube is solid, right? You can see it, feel it, and touch it. If you heat it, it becomes water - fluid. It's a more *subtle* form, but you can still see it, feel it, and touch it.

If you heat the water, it becomes vapor. You can barely see water vapor. It is an even *more subtle* form of energy, and you can barely feel it at all. You may be able to touch it, but it's even less solid than water, isn't it?

But each of these things—the ice, the water, and the vapor—is made of the exact same components.

Okay ... so stick with me here:

Your body is like the ice cube. It's dense, solid, and physical.

But surrounding your body, there is a subtle, invisible field of energy and information: the Biofield. The Biofield comprises your thoughts, feelings, and emotions (which are energy and information too... just more subtle forms of energy. They're like the water and water vapor, when your body is like the ice cube). Your Biofield carries the imprinted vibrational information of everything that's ever happened to you.

Here's something that blew my mind when I realized it:

The subtle creates the physical. In other words, the subtle comes first.

Your thoughts create feelings, and your feelings cause chemical reactions in your body. These chemical reactions affect *everything*, including your organs, your nervous system and immune system.

For example, think about the phrase, "scared myself sick." Perhaps you've experienced this for yourself, when something or someone frightened you so much, you immediately felt sick - literally ill. I know I have experienced this numerous times in my life ... becoming sick with full blown fever, chills, stomach aches, headaches, flu-like symptoms... all of which started with *feeling* afraid.

This demonstrates the power of the strong connection between the mind, the emotions, and the physical symptoms in the body.

When thoughts and feelings are repeated, they create patterns, which can become deeply ingrained just like wearing a groove in a tire. Sometimes these patterns are created quickly, and sometimes they're created slowly, but they stay with us and end up expressing themselves physically in some way, shape, or form.

This understanding of how emotions affect your health is not new. Eastern medicine has long focused on the connection between emotions and health.

Remember, according to the American Psychological Association, two thirds of all Americans said they were likely to seek help for stress. Signs and symptoms of stress include fatigue, headaches, upset stomach, muscle tension, changes in appetite, insomnia, teeth grinding, changes in sex drive, dizziness, irritability, anger, nervousness, lack of energy, and crying.

In our society, "stress" is a word we throw around easily and freely, and it is often simply a *generic term for fear*. It's typically an experience, a *feeling* that you don't like or don't want, so you start to *resist* it.

You may experience a fear of something or someone, or of a particular event, but you refer to it as "stress." Or perhaps something in your current life reminds you of an event or person from your past that was unpleasant, traumatic, fearful, or again, "stressful." Stress (fear) is often the result of your *reactions* to these people, places, and events (current and/or past). Most importantly, it's a result of your *thinking*.

In many cases, stress (fear) comes from imagining the worst and telling yourself a scary story about something in the future that hasn't even happened yet (and this is often based upon what *has* happened to you, in the past).

When the perceived stress occurs, there is an immediate response in the mind, emotions, and the body. Think of this response like an alarm, or a "red alert" going off. The alarm goes off in the mind first, and generates an emotional response, which **then** shows up in the body.

If stress continues, the body then goes into a pattern of adapting to the new, higher level of stress. This increased stress level becomes the new "normal." If the stress continues, it may lead to exhaustion and many other symptoms.

This pattern—alert, adapt, exhaustion, more stress—causes continued mental, emotional, and physical reactions, which continue to send signals to the body, imprinting a pattern of dis-ease which may lead to chronic pain and/or illness.

These thoughts and feelings are energy. They are not separate from your body. Your body is the "outpicturing," the physical expression of your thoughts and feelings.

The real root reason thousands of people are living with chronic pain and stress every single day is that they have never examined the underlying thoughts and emotions that lie beneath the surface and cause that pain and *stress. **They notice the end result and call it "stress." They notice an uncomfortable physical reaction.** **They start to resist it, try to stop it, get rid of it, ignore it, distract themselves from it, suppress and repress it, drug it out or cut it out, or totally deny it altogether, until it gets so uncomfortable, it can no longer be ignored.***

Sound familiar?

If it does, you're one of many who have not been taught to see how your conscious and UN-conscious thoughts and emotional patterns are actually creating and perpetuating the very pain and suffering you're trying to get rid of. AND, to make matters worse, our current culture, educational system, and many religions reinforce certain false and detrimental beliefs such as, "Crying shows weakness," or, "It's unprofessional to get emotional," or, "No pain, no gain," or, "the show must go on, and you must power through no matter how you feel."

These and many other ideas literally keep the stress and pain patterns alive, and practically guarantee that your situation **won't** change one bit!

But I want YOU to know ...

Relief *Is* Possible.

With the right knowledge and the right tools, in the right combination, you CAN experience relief, balance, calm, and even serenity and bliss in your mind, emotions, and body.

If you suffer from chronic pain, depression, anxiety, immune weakness, traumas, digestive disorders, binge-eating, weight issues, and other long-term health challenges, I want you to know that I'm here for YOU. I specialize in helping to *find and release the hidden reasons behind your suffering.*

They're "hidden," because these root causes don't always show up on medical tests, and many well-meaning doctors, healthcare practitioners and even alternative healthcare practitioners haven't been trained to LOOK in the right place for them.

If you've ever heard the words, "'There's nothing we can do for you," or, "You'll just have to cope with this," or, "We have no idea what's causing your pain," then *it's time to change the way **you** think.*

It's time to recognize the deeper level of the symptoms that are expressing in your physical body so you can get your energy and life back on track, so you can do the things you love with the people you love ... and start enjoying life again.

And that's the purpose of this book.

I will continue to share with you not only the insights I've gleaned as I crawled my way out of my own "health hell," but also some actual tools you can use right away to help you begin your journey toward optimum health in a practical, tangible way.

This book has the potential to completely change the direction of your health and your life, starting right now.

If you want that, if you're ready for that, keep reading OR receive my personal help here: **www.BiofieldHealingInstitute.com/dohps**

"You can never cross the ocean until you have the courage to lose sight of the shore."
--- Christopher Columbus

***

My grandfather was born in Russia. As an adult, he decided he wanted a different life for his family. He was opposed to communism, so much so that he decided to exit the country that had always been his "home." He had to "buy" his way out by paying the government a large sum of money, which meant he wasn't able to leave (or start his new life) with any of his hard-earned savings.

He spoke no other language, but his intention to create freedom and his desire to eliminate mental and emotional pain, drove him to leave everything that was familiar, get on a boat, and travel into completely unknown territory. He was navigating by faith alone, propelled by his desire to be rid of his discomfort, and motivated by a deeper "calling": a greater possibility for a better, freer way of life for himself and his family.

The dream of what **was** possible, however **not yet** visible, was a stronger force than the pain associated with staying at the safe and familiar shore, even though he had no guarantee of success.

He only knew that he wanted more, dreamed of a different life for his children, and was willing to go to any lengths to get it. He did not give up hope.

Instead, he took *Action*…he took his entire family, and together, they got on a boat. With nothing.

He somehow knew a better life would manifest for him, and it did (literally!). After an intermediate few years in Cuba where my father was born, he eventually continued on to the United States. He settled in Ohio, and even though he never learned to speak English, he was able to build a thriving business, buy a home, raise 3 boys, and provide a good education for them all.

He enjoyed a full and rich life and lived into his 90's.

Now, I want to ask you:

Are *you* ready to get on the boat? Are you willing to go all in?

Take the first step into the water, now.

Warning: If you're not really ready to open your mind to getting on that boat, to embracing a new possibility for healing your pain, illness, stress, anxiety, or depression, then this book may not be for you. I urge you, from the bottom of my heart, to simply stay open, as you read.

I'd like to begin now with an exercise to help you become present which sets the foundation for healing to occur.

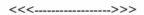

INSTRUCTIONS For This EXERCISE:
Before we get started, an important note about this exercise, and all the exercises that follow: find a safe place to complete the exercises. You should not be driving or operating any equipment or machinery, and I recommend that you practice these sitting up rather than lying down. Some people may experience pressure in the head, slight dizziness, even nausea or other mildly uncomfortable symptoms as they complete these exercises, and even while reading through the book. If this happens to you, please know it's perfectly normal and typically passes rather quickly. It is a sign of healing and simply indicates that you are receiving high vibration, frequencies of healing which I'll discuss in more detail later on in the book.

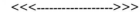

And don't forget - if you really want what I'm sharing with you today to work for you, then you must be fully present and not multi-tasking, especially during the exercises.

Becoming present, just like exercising a new muscle at the gym, gets easier and stronger with practice.

Ready to begin?

Once you've read through the instructions below the first time, complete the exercise with your eyes closed. Know that when you take your attention to your body, and to your breath, you *will* slow down and become more aware. Your mind will follow.

If you ever feel scattered, overwhelmed, confused, anxious, or afraid, or experience any related emotions, just repeat this exercise, to become centered and present. Take deep breaths, and notice how it feels.

EXERCISE: Close your eyes.
- Take a moment right now to just feel your feet on the floor.
- Feel the chair underneath you.
- Now notice the sensation of the air around your face, and pay attention to its temperature and texture as it comes in through your nose.
- Hear the sound of your breath as you exhale.
- Notice the weight of your body and how it feels, as you breathe slowly and deeply through your nose.
- Take your time.
- Breathe deeply and slowly in and out 10 times or more.

Notice yourself becoming more and more present.

Then, when you're ready, move on to Chapter 1.

CHAPTER 1: It ALL Began in Ballet School

Before we dig deep into the hidden reasons you're experiencing pain of some type, and the *revolutionary* healing method that can help, I want you to know that I've been in your shoes.

As the creator of The Pain Free Living Program® and founding director of The Biofield Healing Institute®, I've become known internationally as a pain-release and energy expert, helping people who suffer from a variety of pain symptoms. My unique programs address physical, mental, emotional, and spiritual health, using an effective blend of ancient healing techniques, my own profound method known as Biofield Healing Immersion®, and some of the latest discoveries in physics, neuroscience, and Biofield Science.

I've worked with thousands and thousands of people, all around the globe in over 150 countries, most of whom I've never even met, and every day, I still pinch myself! I've witnessed - and continue to witness - incredible healing results and extraordinary transformations.

Getting to this place has been a long and winding journey, with many hills and valleys, and I believe it all was set in motion when I was just 4 years old, at my ballet school in Cincinnati, Ohio.

I started taking dance lessons because I wanted to be like my beautiful cousin, Elaine. She was popular, graceful, kind, and talented. I admired her so much.

At ballet school, I learned to move and count to the beats of the music, and in retrospect, it's also where my ideal life path began to emerge (although I didn't know it at that time).

Now, years later, I realize that everything I learned about energy healing, I learned in ballet school.

In each class, (although they didn't use this language) we explored how to feel into the space around us, how to see in all directions, and how to connect and communicate - without words - with everyone onstage and in the audience. I learned how to hold everyone, near and far, in my "field of awareness," in my consciousness, aware of them at all times in all locations. I learned how to move through space in any direction, *seeing and feeling with my entire body, mind, emotions, and soul.*

Eyes open, eyes closed … it didn't matter.

I became highly sensitive to the slightest nuance, subtle energetic shifts and changes, and to the existence of a vast amount of information that is present everywhere, that lies both in our bodies and in the invisible energetic field all around us.

You too can become sensitive to this subtle energy and information; however, if you are like most of the people I've worked with and trained in my method, you probably are not aware of this. You may not notice these constant nuances because your analytical mind is filled with way too much "mind-chatter" or your emotions (the ones you don't know how to release) get in the way and cloud over your ability to sense the subtle information that is there all the time. In fact, most thoughts are UN-conscious and come from early childhood conditioning.

Your mind may be so busy with thoughts, and it may seem like they just "happen" to you. Therefore, you may believe you have no ability to change them or quiet them.

The mind is designed to think ... and think ... and think some more. The brain behaves like a search engine, constantly seeking out "like items," or similar thoughts. If you have been, or are currently, around "negative" conversations, a lot of criticism, and/or "upsetting" environments, you may find it difficult to get this off your mind, and eventually, your mind can become filled with constant chatter.

That's how it was for me many times in my life, and I would have given *anything* for some peace and quiet in my head! It was like an endless committee meeting, and the chatter never stopped, and the story it was telling wasn't even any good!

But throughout my dance training, I practiced ways to focus my thinking, quiet my mind, and learned to use my imagination to rehearse the choreography *internally* first, inside my mind's eye, which later caused actual physical improvements in my performance while onstage.

No one called it "creative visualization" back then, but *I was learning to harness the inner powers of thought, using directed focus, imagination and intention.*

Unbeknownst to me at that time, I was training for what has become my highest calling to date—Biofield Healing®.

"Imagination is more powerful than knowledge."
--- *Albert Einstein*

As a child, I had discovered how to go within, and listen inside to the subtle messages my own thoughts, feelings, and body were sending me, as well as all the constant information being communicated around me, from other people and the environment.

I recognized the wisdom, the answers, and the information was *there*, inside of me. And I began to trust it.

Then, when I was 15, my friend Peter came to visit. He told me about his sister, who was initiating people into Transcendental Meditation (also known as TM). I had no idea what he was talking about ... I'd never even heard the word, "meditation."

But the second I heard Peter say, "Transcendental Meditation," I knew I *had* to do it. Every fiber of my being was 100% in, even though I hadn't a clue what I was actually getting into.

I have come to believe that I was actually "coded" for that moment in time. It was intuitive guidance that could not be ignored, even though there was no apparent logical explanation.

I heard "The Call."

I asked my father for the $150 I needed to begin taking the TM course, and to put it mildly, he freaked. He told me it was a cult, and not to mention TM again.

I insisted. I told him it was my destiny. I tried reasoning with him. Peter's sister was a professional. She helped people. She wasn't a high school dropout. Meditation helped people.

Still, my father didn't buy it.

I began to beg, plead, moan, storm, shout, demand, and cry. Hysterically.

That backfired.

He told me that if I **was** mature enough to learn to meditate, I wouldn't be throwing a temper tantrum like a 2-year-old.

But I simply had to learn. I could not, and would not, accept, "No," as an answer. So I got a job, earned the money I needed, and began my studies at the TM Center.

Meditation changed my life, dramatically.

I began to discover an even richer inner world, filled with unique information, and experiences.

I took the practice of meditation very seriously. I hung a sign on my bedroom door twice daily, that clearly stated, "Do not disturb for any reason. I am meditating."

No one in my family respected the sign, but that didn't stop me. I endured the interruptions, and practiced learning to drop beneath the "noise," to stay present, to allow and observe even when things didn't go as I wished during my sacred meditation time.

Through this daily practice, *I developed an even deeper awareness of subtle energy,* states of consciousness different from the normal waking state. I tapped into feelings of peace and calm and even bliss that were in complete contrast to my "regular" life.

Meditation literally saved me from some of the turmoil and constant fighting that occurred in my family during my teenage years. It connected me to "something greater", to "something higher," to a state of calm and helped me become less reactionary.

This "something"—the mystery—became my daily friend, and I was fascinated by the journey within.

Fast-forward: I left college early, leaving Arizona State University's Dance Department my senior year before even utilizing the dance scholarship I'd been awarded. I moved to New York City to live my dream after being hired to dance professionally with an Off-Broadway modern dance company. I thought I had died and gone to heaven!

The opportunity opened with such ease and grace. It was a dancer's dream-come-true. Algebra could wait! All of those years of sore muscles, learning to spin on one leg, and walking like a duck were finally paying off.

I simply HAD to go.

Before I knew it, I was dancing professionally in what I considered the greatest city on earth. I had the opportunity to study with some of the world's finest choreographers including Merce Cunningham and Viola Farber, and was awarded a full scholarship at Alvin Ailey Dance Theatre. My dreams were coming true!

It *was* an amazing opportunity, but after years being immersed in the lifestyle, I realized it was anything but glamorous. Bloody feet, exhaustion, hunger, no personal life, fierce physical demands, constant stress, and fierce competition were my regular, and often only, companions. Sure, as dancers, we smiled on stage … but backstage, it was a completely different story.

I endured multiple technique classes 6 days per week, long rehearsals, and frequent performances for little-to-no wages. I spent many days and nights in dingy rehearsal halls and theatres, often with no heat. I waited tables on the side, just so I could survive.

The whole time, I couldn't help but hear my father's voice, proclaiming over and over that this dancing career was a bad decision, and nothing good could come of it.

One day I just couldn't take it anymore. The choreography was particularly brutal that season and involved a lot of falling (on purpose) and being thrown (on purpose) and being draped over props made of metal. I literally was black and blue with bruises all over my body from these rehearsals.

I woke up one morning and knew I simply could not go on. I remember as if it was yesterday; I called my father crying, in desperate need of support and encouragement.

He said, "When are you going to get a real job?"

So I quit. That day. End of story.

I ended my dance career with my dad's words ringing in my ears and set out to get a "real" job.

Thus began what I refer to as "The Corporate Chapter."

My humble beginning was not glamorous in this world either, but I was used to pain, and I had to start somewhere.

The very next day I called a well-known Manhattan employment agency. They asked me what my previous professional work experience was.

I said, "Modern Dancer."

They hung up on me. (No joke!)

Determined to get a job, I called right back and confidently declared, "I can *type*!"

That actually did the trick and got me an interview, which lead to the "real" job. This was my introduction into the corporate world. Of course, I was placed at the bottom rung of every ladder and pay scale, and treated accordingly.

It was a huge challenge to say the least, and I felt like a fish out of water.

After being a dancer my whole life, I was miserable behind a desk. Everyone around me seemed content sitting all day, eating candy, and counting the hours until TGIF and happy hour came along.

I was NOT content.

Although I was learning some new, great, useful skills, I felt lost. I constantly questioned my choices and the direction of my life, and I had no idea where I was headed or how the current chapter I was living would end. I certainly didn't have a life plan. Goals? No. I had none.

I basically wandered aimlessly, trying to mimic the plans and values of others, hoping my "real" job would somehow lead to happiness.

Dancing had been my only real passion up to that point, and it seemed nothing could replace it.

Eating a lot of ice cream and drinking alcohol turned out to be the best solution I could come up with at the time, and helped to numb my pain and quiet the mind chatter I mentioned earlier. I had no support and told no one about my feelings. Instead, I just kept wishing and hoping that somehow things would magically lead to happiness.

A few years later, New York had lost its luster. It just seemed cold, ugly, and expensive. I wanted a change.

I blamed my unhappiness *on* New York … and at that time in my life I didn't understand one important truth:

You take yourself with you wherever you go.

Making a geographical change may lead to a temporary "honeymoon" phase, but if you don't take a good hard look at yourself and change yourself on the *inside*—your consciousness, your thinking, and your actions—then, eventually, the patterns just repeat, no matter where you are.

Because I didn't realize this yet, I decided I'd move to California. I had often dreamed of living by the ocean, and I thought, confidently, *that* would solve my unhappiness.

What was supposed to be a short stop in Arizona (to see an old boyfriend) derailed my California-or-Bust plan (that's a story for a whole separate book!), and I ended up staying in Arizona for much longer than I originally anticipated.

Little did I know at that time in my life that *everything* has a reason, a higher purpose, and this unplanned, new road would lead me right to the doorstep of a grand awakening and transformation.

Through repeating my painful patterns of running away, avoiding, stuffing, denying, numbing out feelings, fantasy thinking and much more, I would eventually wake myself up and discover the secrets to happiness I had been searching for my entire life.

In that hot desert where most things that are planted have little chance of surviving and growing, the next chapter of my life was born, and I, Debora Wayne, the *real* me, began to blossom.

In the desert, I found myself, but not without a very "dark night of the soul."

On the outside, things started looking better immediately…I found a new "real" job, a new relationship, and put some money in the bank (do you see the pattern here of "everything starts out great", beginning again?).

But I (the real me, inside) had not changed one bit, and over time, I began to experience a tsunami of pain building up again. I wasn't happy. Things weren't going as planned. The thrill of the new job and new relationship started wearing off.

I didn't see where my life was headed. I couldn't seem to fill that empty hole inside no matter how much money I made or material possessions I acquired. Something was still missing. I felt lost, filled with a horrible loneliness and sense of hopelessness most of the time.

Once again, I followed the same formula of pretending, fantasy thinking, not finding my own passions, ignoring and going against my values, and not following my intuition at all.

I desperately tried to be good enough, smart enough, pretty enough, and perfect enough to please everyone else.

I kept trying harder, giving more, working longer hours, getting more degrees, buying new clothes, taking vacations, purchasing more stuff, trying to be nicer, be tougher … attempting to control, control, control both myself and others.

Nothing seemed to work, and I was becoming increasingly frustrated and exhausted!

I became depressed. I was anxious and full of fear. I drank more and more in an attempt to alleviate those uncomfortable feelings, just to get through each day. I continued wishing and hoping things would somehow magically change.

My mind was never peaceful. The negative voices never shut up. I kept all my thoughts and fears bottled up inside and chanted my favorite mantra: "Everything is fine," "Everything is fine," "Everything is fine."

But it wasn't fine—*at all!*

I started to experience a lot of physical pain and symptoms. My hair was falling out, I had constant headaches, stomach aches, insomnia, severe PMS, low thyroid, adrenal exhaustion, "mysterious" aches and pains that would come and go, constant cravings for sweets, extraordinary fatigue, and more.

I felt bored… Flat… Apathetic… Nervous… Edgy… Irritable… Impatient. Depression flip-flopped with Anxiety. It took a lot of energy to shove all these feelings underground, and eventually I began to lose touch with how I was feeling entirely.

"I just need a little vacation," I would tell myself. "It's just stress! No big deal."

But it *was* a big deal, and I was ignoring all the signs.

I was spiraling more and more deeply into my own personal health hell. Each day became increasingly difficult to power through. There wasn't enough alcohol, pot, pills, designer shoes, or Ben and Jerry's ice cream to numb all the pain, and I found myself in that same dark place I'd been in before I left New York.

Something had to change. *I couldn't live like this one more day.*

I remember it clearly. I was sitting in the dark, on the floor. I couldn't get dressed, I couldn't stop crying, and I couldn't go to work. I couldn't move.

I just sat there sobbing on the floor of my beautiful, perfect walk-in closet that housed all of my perfect clothes, in my perfect house, in our perfect neighborhood, while my perfect husband was at his perfect job.

We had everything: the house, a BMW in the garage, custom-tailored clothes, modern furnishings, plenty of food in the fridge.

But inside, I was empty. Bankrupt.

And I was *sick*. My hair was falling out; I had ulcers and a thyroid condition; and as I mentioned previously, a slew of other painful symptoms.

I couldn't sleep through the night, unless, of course, I drank a lot of wine and popped a few of those "non-addicting" sedatives.

Fear began to consume me. I became afraid of everything: other people, what people thought about me, being seen, speaking up, telling the truth, being wrong, being successful, failing, looking stupid, making mistakes, love, responsibility, having no money, having too much money, gaining weight ... afraid of bread, sugar, coffee, oil, butter, meat, salt, hurting someone's feelings, traveling, being "stuck," getting lost, the unknown, being bored ... afraid of death, afraid of life...I was afraid of it all!

You get it. Fear, fear, fear was completely taking over!

I had no idea this fear was causing severe symptoms in my physical body. I had no idea it was causing the mysterious pains that came and went, but never showed up on medical tests.

I had followed the "formula for happiness" and couldn't figure out the answer to the all-encompassing question: *Why do I still hurt?*

By some miracle, on this day, the day I found myself on the floor of my closet, knowing something had to change, I stopped. That time, instead of running, instead of blaming everyone and everything else...for once, I actually stopped.

I stopped everything and finally asked for help.

I uttered a desperate prayer: "God, help me."

I was a nervous wreck but somehow, an unfamiliar sense of courage came over me and I reached for the phone book, called a total stranger, and asked this professional for help. This day was a major turning point in my life and it proved to be the greatest decision I could have ever made.

I found myself very shortly thereafter entering an entirely new world of personal and spiritual growth. I joined a group program and learned how to get radically honest with myself and others about my feelings. I began to receive quality, unconditional love and support, as well as numerous new tools that I desperately needed. I finally learned how to end the Blame Game, to stop giving my power away, and to stop running away from problems. I changed the entire course of my life. I was finally, with the aid of great support, able and willing to find my own truth and start getting my life back on the right track.

Getting help gave me the proper guidance and courage to be able to look *within myself*, the proper tools to face my inner demons and finally find answers and peace.

I learned that pain is a blessing in disguise. It's trying to get our attention for a reason, and it is not to be ignored. Whether it's physical, mental, emotional, spiritual, financial, or any kind of pain whatsoever, it must come up, in order for it to move out. Pain is a blessing in disguise. Always.

Things began changing quickly in my life, and it wasn't all smooth and easy sailing by any means. My husband and I agreed to a separation. I moved out of my perfect house into a tiny condo, taking only a chair and blanket with me.

At first, I was so out of touch with myself that I didn't even know what I liked to eat. I had a closet full of clothes I didn't feel comfortable in because they weren't "me" and didn't fit.

I got honest with myself and realized I'd chosen the career I had found myself "stuck" in to impress my father ... it wasn't even something I had enjoyed. At the same time, I didn't have the confidence to try anything new.

The day before Easter Sunday, 1984, I was alone and feeling rather miserable, swimming in a sea of self-pity. I sat staring at the blank, white walls of my furniture-less, tiny condo, when I felt something stir inside me.

It was anger. Here I was **again**... starting over *again* with nothing and no one.

I walked out onto my third-floor patio and looked over the railing to the drop below. It was a long drop.

The night sky was pitch black. I knew no one could see me.

I held onto the railing so tightly my fingers turned colors, and then I did it: I screamed, at the top of my lungs, "If there's a God, I need proof! Where are you? Who are you? Are you there? Is anyone there? I need your help!"

Then, quite surprisingly, help arrived yet again, but this time in a more dramatic fashion that is unforgettable to this day.

I don't know where it came from, but I undeniably received it.

I was flooded with the most divine feeling of total peace, engulfed in a clearly palpable cosmic cocoon of unconditional love and bliss.

A beacon of white light beamed straight down from the full moon. It surrounded the entire patio and bathed me in that abyss of unconditional love.

The next thing I knew, communication took place. This was not an audible voice, but a direct "knowing"... A telepathic, silent communication that I could hear nonetheless.

I knew absolutely without a shadow of a doubt that everything was going to be all right.

I relaxed.

My entire body relaxed for the first time in years.

There was no more pain, no more head chatter, and no more critical inner voice. There was only silence and the expansive feeling of unconditional love.

It was incredible and unexplainable.

From that moment in time, I found myself filled with passion and energy, with clear life-direction.

In Phoenix, Arizona rising from the ashes, the real Debora was reborn, and I finally began to really heal from the inside out.

I began to see and feel real change and real progress.   I began to honor my own unique life path, and to experience receiving clear guidance from within on a daily basis. Life became more effortless and began to flow with greater ease.   I felt hopeful and positive and excited about the future. I found a new sense of courage and was able to take risks, try new things, meet new people and move beyond my comfort zone like never before.

The healing occurred first on the inside, but the physical followed shortly after. My energy came back in spades! People commented that I looked 10 years younger, and I could feel it!

I went back to school and a new career path began to unfold. I found myself eager to learn again. I devoured book after book, discovered spiritual support groups, yoga classes, salsa dancing, took art classes, and spent quiet time every single day in nature and meditation, seeking my own personal truth. The path began to reveal itself to me one step at a time.

I learned for the first time that I was not my title. I learned it was okay to *be* myself and not try to prove my worth by *doing* and over-giving. I experienced living in the moment, trusting the process, and enjoying the entire daily journey not just the end goal.

I went from having zero energy and zero passion to being totally filled with vitality, ideas, and enthusiasm for so many new things I could hardly do them all!

First, I discovered a strong interest in the Healing Arts and immersed myself in the subject, earning degrees and certifications in psychology, hypnotherapy, and chemical dependency counseling. I returned to my daily meditation practice and became a certified yoga instructor and a Reiki Master. I read everything I could get my hands on regarding spiritual healing and paranormal psychology.

Time was flying by, and I felt happy and peaceful - like I was finally on the right track. Within what felt like no time, I was teaching, working in treatment centers with adults and teenagers, and seeing private clients. I facilitated women's groups and introduced foreign ingredients like Hypnotherapy and NLP into my work. At the time, these were very cutting edge, and few people knew what these tools were.

"Stress management" was just gaining recognition as an important ingredient for achieving good health, and it was relatively novel to discuss how our thinking might be related to pain, problems, and symptoms.

I was even more excited about the results I was seeing from practicing spiritual healing techniques (today we might call it energy healing). Although I was thrilled about this, I was still quietly tiptoeing around the fact that I had discovered the ability to use my hands working directly with life-force energy for the purpose of healing.

I found that I was able to help people de-stress, to release pain, tension, and undesirable emotions, and to quiet their disturbed minds without the use of drugs or mood-altering chemicals.

Peace and healing became my new calling.

I also reunited with my inner artist and unleashed her! I went back to ceramics classes, dabbled in handmade paper, and started working in glass. Something, some big energy took over. The life force inside me when I connected to the creative flow was incredible. I jumped out of bed each morning, eager and excited to experiment, create, and see what I'd be taught *from within.*

I began to see my life puzzle fitting together. The visual arts, like dance and meditation, helped me to refine my sensitivities to the subtle and not-so-subtle energies I could harness for the purpose of helping others heal and to affect environments in a positive way.

The process of creating mesmerized me.

I tapped into an unlimited source of creativity and energy, and experienced an unlimited flow of ideas. I recognized this potential unfurling inside myself. I used all my new tools to let go of the critical voices and simply allow artistic expression to come through me without censorship.

What ensued was extraordinary.

With no savings account whatsoever, no support from friends or family, a Visa card with only a $1000 limit, and no formal art education, I went from mere experimentation to developing a HIGH 6-figure business in less than one year!

By simply discovering how to tap into my intuition and develop a strong connection to the creative Source, I was able to open a retail storefront in downtown Scottsdale and a showroom for the interior design trade, and to sell my works in glass to more than 500 wholesale and retail accounts including fine art galleries, museum shops, and specialty gift stores all across the US.

I was pinching myself. How could it possibly get any better than this?

Yet it does.

Remember that dream I had, to live in California?

Well, that dream finally came true as I followed my heart and guidance, and in 2006, I entered the next life-changing chapter, which further defined my path.

Everything lined up. It became perfectly clear that it was finally time ... time to leave the desert and move to the ocean. Within less than 4 weeks, my Arizona home was rented, my art studio and office were sublet, and I had a fantastic new art studio, office, and residence lined up in California just 3 blocks from the Pacific Ocean.

31

Joyous is an understatement when it comes to describing moving day. Even my movers had fun!

Shortly after moving to California, I was invited to co-teach a Yoga workshop and offer Reiki Sessions in Hawaii.

You have to understand that I had been facilitating Reiki healing sessions pretty much in secret for years. Only my yoga students and certain friends knew about this. Although I'd seen the "proof" of my ability to facilitate some results, I was never really sure whether it was myself, or God, or angels at work. Because of my doubt-heavy mindset, I lacked confidence, so I never fully stepped into this area of the work in a visible or more public way.

I worried: What if nothing happened? What if I wasn't doing it right? What will people think?

The results from Reiki were often very subtle. People would say the sessions were "relaxing," and I always told myself that of course it was relaxing to lie down for an hour. I wasn't really sure if I was actually helping my clients in any tangible, "real" way.

Back to Hawaii, 2006: I agreed to teach the yoga workshop and was about to begin the very first Reiki session with one of the students who happened to be someone I had never met before. We were in a beautiful outdoor setting on the back lawn of a private plantation on Kona. Who wouldn't be relaxed? Birds singing, grass smelling divine, flowers, fruit trees ... so perfectly quiet.

I went to begin the Reiki session, raised my hands, and all of a sudden, *I gasped as I heard the silence speak.*

It was another unexpected divine moment.

I held my breath in. I couldn't exhale. I heard the silent words I'll never forget ... and a deep knowing came with it:

"You're done with Reiki. Stand still and just let it flow through you."

Someone, something, some mysterious force turned on the faucet. Energy started *pouring* out of my hands. It was electric, palpable, intense, like nothing I'd ever felt before. For the first time, I absolutely, 100 percent *knew* it was not me doing this. This was clearly a power much greater than myself.

There was no questioning this.

Even my mind chatter came to a halt.

There was calm, quiet, and most importantly, a knowing that this was real.

This mysterious force continued to flow through my hands with full strength.

Eventually I brought the session to a close. Ann still hadn't spoken or moved for more than an hour.

For a moment, I was concerned about what her reaction would be as I helped her sit up. But I knew something BIG had happened. I knew it wasn't me causing this electricity, this energy.

It came through me, but it was not ME generating it.

When Ann opened her eyes, she said to me: "That was the most profound experience I've ever had. I've carried tremendous physical and emotional pain for the past 20+ years. I now know it was the result of unresolved conflicts I had with my mother who died ten years ago. During our session I made complete peace with her and everything upsetting that occurred between us. It was like a high-speed movie flashing before my eyes. All the pain and issues between us became clear as day. I felt it all, but it wasn't painful. I released it all. I communicated with my mother and I heard her speak back to me. We made peace. I feel free. My physical and emotional pain is gone now. I know I will never be the same, and I cannot thank you enough."

Shock.

This was the birthday of the Biofield Healing Immersion ® method.

And I couldn't wait to do it again.

Of course, the inevitable mind chatter piped up, but I persevered.

And guess what?

This remarkable healing experience, which helped Ann become pain free and brought her, in her own words, "bliss, joy, and peace," has happened again and again and again, innumerable times since that first time on Kona.

I've since had the incredible opportunity to work with tens of thousands of people all over the globe, who have reported the elimination of chronic pain, depression, anxiety, trauma, immune disorders, and numerous other painful patterns and conditions as a result of this powerful and effective modality, Biofield Healing Immersion®.

Want to experience this for yourself? Join me here:
www.BiofieldHealingInstitute.com/dohps

I am still excited, shocked, curious, thrilled, humbled, and pinching myself, daily, at the transformations I am privileged to witness and be part of.

That's why I wrote this book.

To give you hope, and make **you** aware of something you most likely do not know exists that may help you and be the answer you've been searching for and praying for.

Biofield Healing Immersion® is a truly revolutionary method that has the potential to rapidly remove your pain, restore your energy, and get your life back on the right track.

"I experienced a profound healing from Fibromyalgia with Debora Wayne. After 20 years of symptomatic pain, I could feel the sources of this auto-immune disorder being pulled from my body during her session."
--- *Maryanne, San Diego, CA*

"Debora's power was so great! I had **Chronic Fatigue** and guess what? It's gone!!"
--- *Helen, Ichikawa, Japan*

***

Biofield Healing Immersion® may help **you** finally find inner peace, get your joy back, experience ease and comfort physically, mentally, emotionally, and feel a deep connection to your intuition, to nature, to other people, to yourself, and to the entire cosmos. It truly has the potential to be life-changing for you.

***

"A life-altering process…Debora put me in a state of bliss. This has been more powerful for me than any other modality I have been exposed to…significantly higher. It definitely changed my level of consciousness dramatically."
--- *Gregg, La Jolla, CA*

***

With Biofield Healing Immersion® beneficial results are often achieved effortlessly and rapidly, sometimes occurring even by participating in just a short demonstration session. Most people have an experience that they know is "real" and cannot deny. This is not an intellectual process and does not require you to believe in anything or even understand Biofield Healing Immersion® with your mind.

***

"My shoulder was pain free after the session. This was a "real" experience something I can believe is real and seems very different to my experiences in my everyday world. I feel restored."

"I am able to feel in my body, and the pressure in my head and jaw also released."
--- *Mary Green, Australia*

"After my second Biofield Healing session....I woke up in the morning and I had no more pain! I came out of my shell and I was full of energy, vibrancy, and life! It was amazing."
---*Steve*

"My Asthma is entirely gone after only one session with Debora."
---*Suzy H. San Diego, CA*

***

Even practitioners, who typically have experienced numerous other alternative methods of healing all say the same thing:
    Wow, This is different! This is incredible!'

***

"Working with Debra I immediately felt relief from mental pain. My body was lighter and my mind clearer.

Within 24 hours of my first Biofield Healing Immersion® session, I felt physical pain and emotional pain leave my body.

I am a changed person. Everything has changed in my life. I am excited about my future and so very grateful for the healing I have received."
---*Sharon Henderson, NV*

"I have had two knee operations and a 2 inch plate implanted in my neck. I have been in constant pain for years - since 2000.

I was skeptical. I was totally surprised at the response of my body to Debora's Biofield Healing Immersion® method.

Remember, I had already tried everything - Acupuncture, Acupressure, and all types of other physical treatments. Nothing had ever felt like this.
I felt so good after the Biofield Healing Immersion® session. There was relief from pain showing in my face, and my attitude was now more optimistic.

I don't have to take pain medication or muscle relaxers any longer. I haven't felt this good in years! This spiritual healing from Debora Wayne, is real.
I was healed from the inside out. It lasts , it works, and the only side effect is better health. THANK YOU"
---*Louis, Orange, CA*

I have an MS diagnosis and disability due to injuries from an assault.

I listened to your recording, and WOW! 'THANK YOU! Thank you, Debora Wayne for the fact that I could just walk into my kitchen - with crutches - but I WALKED!

Over the last few hours, pain is being released as years of trauma are freed and released. I have worked with doctors and therapists using CPT, DBT, EFT, EMDR, and PE to process and release trauma with little effect on my physical condition.

WHY DO I STILL HURT?

As a PhD holding chemical physicist, I have known the pain is energetic in origin, but have not been able to address it alone... Until Now"
---*Gail Marlow, Ph.D - University Chemistry Professor (former)*

***

The possibilities are endless and the results often so exciting I simply have to share this with the world.

I've practiced, researched, and facilitated thousands and thousands of sessions, one-on-one, online, in groups, and even via Mp3 recordings. I've worked with people all over the entire world, many of whom I'm never met or even spoken to and people keep reporting incredible results.

***

"I was losing my life, it was over. Then...through Debora, I got my life back. No other words. A miracle. "
--- *CiCi, Encinitas, CA*

"In 6 short weeks I went from massive back pain and living in a residence that I disliked.... to packing over 100 boxes and moving into a wonderful new place! And all while working at a demanding job!

... the change is remarkable and undeniable.

Looking forward to more of that lovely Biofield Healing®!"
-----*YC, Technical Writer, Calgary, AB, Canada*

"My skeleton realigned itself after our Distance Session just like when I've had hands on treatment. That's incredible...remote energy work that realigned my spine!!! Even my ankles are realigned. My back has felt great ever since the first session. The way a back should feel. My neck, shoulder, and low back pain are all gone."
---*Jim J., Simi Valley, CA*

Are you excited to discover and EXPERIENCE more for yourself?

I hope so!

If you are ready right now to jump in and begin *YOUR* personal experience of Biofield Healing Immersion® ...
If you'd like to discover the hidden root causes of your pain and suffering (that don't show up on medical tests) and Release them...
If you'd like to *finally* stop the pain of trying to figure out what's wrong and how to get your pain to stop...
If you'd like to remove your pain, restore and recharge your energy, and get your life back on track...
If you want to discover the 3 EXACT things you must do if you want to learn to live pain free...

Then please accept my help and BEGIN RIGHT NOW to experience this incredible method for yourself. www.BiofieldHealingInstitute.com/dohps

Next, I'd like you to complete the following exercise, which I've designed to help you get the most out of reading the remainder of this book.

INSTRUCTIONS For This EXERCISE:
Remember: find a safe place to complete the exercises. You should not be driving or operating any equipment or machinery, and it's best to do this sitting up rather than lying down. Some people may experience pressure in the head, slight dizziness, even nausea or other mildly uncomfortable symptoms as they complete these exercises, and even while reading through the book. If this happens to you, please know it's perfectly normal and indicates that you are receiving and responding to frequencies of healing. These are higher vibrations than you are used to and the discomfort normally passes quickly. Just breathe, relax, and allow them to integrate.

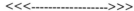

EXERCISE –
"Shift From Impossible to Possible"

Take a moment right now to open your mind to new possibilities.

Close your eyes and envision a large whiteboard in front of you with the word "Impossible" written on it.

Now imagine a giant eraser.

Imagine the eraser easily, quickly, and *immediately* wiping off the word, "Impossible."

Wipe the board completely clean.

Now imagine a new phrase appearing on the whiteboard: "All things are possible!"

As you see this on the whiteboard also *feel* into it.

Next, imagine a doorway at the top of your head, and open that door wide open.

Imagine the sentence, "All Things Are Possible," literally floating off the whiteboard and flowing in through the top of your head.

Feel how your mind is now open.

Remember...I am not trying to convince you of anything nor take anything away from you either. Just be open to some new ideas and new ways of thinking, feeling, acting, and being. Be open to ideas and concepts that you may not understand yet, but that may become your new truth. Realize that you don't HAVE to understand every bit of what I share with you today for this to help you get positive results ... just be *open* and curious, whether you fully understand or not. Experiment with the exercises throughout this book and try on these new concepts and see for yourself what happens.

Lift your chest and sit up tall now and take a deep breath—a really deep breath—and exhale while saying the words, "I am open. I am open to receiving. I am open and I know and trust that everything I need to know will be revealed to me in the perfect right way at the perfect right time."

Sit quietly for a moment, and to the best of your ability simply notice, feel, observe, and allow whatever you are experiencing right now to be OK - without making any judgment.

When you're ready, move on to Chapter 2

CHAPTER 2: Some Fundamental Truths About the Universe and *You*

You're going to hear me say this again and again:

You can't separate your body from your mind or your emotions ... and you can't separate your body, mind, and emotions from your spirit.

Your *natural* state IS a state of health and wholeness and peace.

And your body never lies. So if you're experiencing pain, anxiety, or depression, it's time to learn fundamental truths about yourself, what dis-ease is, and where it really comes from.

It's time to explore the body, the mind, the emotions, and the spirit at the quantum level: the energetic level.

***

Your body, your mind, and your emotions are the doorways to discovering the root cause of all your stress and pain (we'll talk more about these doorways in the next chapter).

Your Inner Environment Is Essentially Causing Your Physical Reality.

It's been my experience that most people don't realize their thoughts and emotions are contributing to their pain and suffering. They haven't been taught how powerful thoughts are, or how buried emotions cause harm. Most people I work with tell me they think their thoughts and feelings "just happen" ... a mysterious process.

But it isn't mysterious at all. Let me explain.

You see, the body is a metaphor for our consciousness ... it is the "outpicturing," the physical expression of what is going on in the mind, emotions, and in your life, and it's here to teach you, to help you learn things that you *need* to learn.

Everything is energy ... including your physical body.
All thoughts and all feelings are subtle energy, and the subtle energetic level creates the physical.

Everything begins at the subtle level and becomes physical, not the other way around.

(Pause for a moment and really let that sink in.)

Think about the chair you sit on. Before it became a physical object, it was *first* a thought in someone's mind. It didn't just appear out of thin air.

Without realizing this important point, that thoughts and feelings are the pre-cursor to the physical, you embody the role of "victim, "with seemingly no control over your own personal state of health.

Maybe it seems like illness and pain happen for no reason - like everything is happening by chance or coincidence. Perhaps you've learned to blame your genetics. This type of thinking keeps you trapped; when you don't understand what is happening to you, and when you don't have solutions to change these things, you experience even more stress and anxiety, which lead to more pain and symptoms. Then, you're stuck in a continuous, never-ending downward spiral, as your physical, mental, and emotional health deteriorate.

In reality, we have thoughts all the time *about* people, *about* situations, and *about* events that occur. In fact, science has proven that on average, we think 50,000-60,000 thoughts per day. Many of these are not positive or pleasant thoughts.

Thoughts *cause* feelings. And feelings cause chemical reactions in your body. These chemical reactions, in turn, affect your nervous system, your immune system, even specific organs that affect your overall state of health.

Many of these thoughts aren't even true, but we take them to heart as if they are ("I'm not good enough," "I'm not smart enough," "No one cares about me" … all those negative thoughts you've likely believed at some point in the your life).

And you know when this is happening. You can *feel* it, and you know that something is wrong. You may try to control these feelings by asking yourself **why** you're thinking certain thoughts, and then attempting to **stop** yourself from doing so. You may try to get rid of them in some way, and start to resist, deny, suppress, or repress them, thinking it will bring relief…but it never does.

When feelings and thoughts are repeated (whether they are true or not) and not properly resolved and released in the natural way they're designed to, they create patterns of tension, stress, and discomfort. The original thoughts and feelings that created these patterns often become buried deep down, hidden from view, yet they show up later as physical "symptoms" of pain and dis-ease. Thoughts and feelings are constantly communicating energetically with the cells of your body, literally creating your physical reality. Your biofield holds all of this information and is the key to both health **and** dis-ease.

You may feel stuck and blocked, and worse, scared that you'll never find relief.

This—the unexpressed, unacknowledged, and unreleased negative thoughts, feelings, and all the energy from past traumas and events remain lingering with and affecting you after they have long since passed. This is the #1 culprit hidden from your view when it comes to dis-ease.

I've experienced this on my own health journey, and also found this to be true with 99.99% of the clients, students, and practitioners with whom I've worked or trained.

I have found after many years of working with people of all ages and with all forms of illness that once the mental and emotional patterns are discovered and properly released, the "physical conditions" often naturally dissolve and disappear ... and oftentimes, this happens instantaneously!

That's the great news!

The thing is, your biofield is like a video recorder that is turned on 24/7, recording every moment from your entire life—creating imprints of experiences from as early on as the womb, childhood, young adulthood and adulthood. These imprints remain in your field. Feelings you denied, suppressed, repressed, or never fully felt also linger in your biofield, and may be affecting your health in a negative way. They're imprints of things you've learned, things you've picked up from other people, your environment ... everything! These imprints can continue to operate for years, stuck on autopilot, creating patterns in your emotional and physical state.

That's the bad news, but don't worry ... because there *is* a solution!

All of the answers you seek can be accessed inside of you. Your thoughts, your feelings, and your body can give you clues to the real root cause of your physical symptoms, and your body is designed to heal itself.

"New-edge science reveals that our power to control our lives originates from our minds, and is not preprogrammed in our genes. To activate the amazing power of mind over genes, we must reconsider our fundamental beliefs - our perceptions and misperceptions- of life."
---Bruce Lipton, Ph.D.

Let's talk about quantum physics for a moment (for those of you who appreciate the science!). Quantum physics is basically the study of how energy works. Quantum Theory says that *everything* is made up of energy. Studies and research have proven this theory.

- Everything in the Universe is made up of subatomic particles (think electrons) that exist as Pure Potential in a waveform state.
- They are so small they are hardly measurable.
- Matter, on the subatomic level, exists as a momentary phenomenon.
- The particles are so small, they are almost non-existent. They appear and disappear into 3 dimensions and back into the field in no space, no time, transforming from particle (matter) to wave (energy).
- The person observing the particles affects the behavior of the atoms.
- Energy responds to your mindful attention and BECOMES matter.

In other words, our thoughts affect energy AND physical matter.

* Note: *This theory dates back to the 1800s, and was influenced by scientists including Albert Einstein, Michael Faraday, Gustav Kirchoff, Ludwig Boltzmann, Heinrich Hertz, Max Planck, Max Born, Werner Heisenberg, and Wolfgang Pauli.*

In the mid-1980's, Russian scientists defined the existence of an additional class of fields (we're talking about physics here) beyond the 4 types known at that time: gravitational, electrical, magnetic, and nuclear.

The new field type they discovered is often referred to as a "spin field," a "torsion field," or an "information field." As the name indicates, these fields are filled not just with energy, but also with information.

[* Source:.] **Torsion: A "Fifth Force" Synonymous with Consciousness? --Brendan D. Murphy**

Your thoughts, the thoughts of others, and the world around you constantly communicate information via your field. As I understand it, your field is basically continuously recording and communicating, and if you don't know how to properly release the "disturbed" information specifically in relation to pain, trauma, false beliefs etc., they linger in your field and affect you. They create disturbance patterns, and then finally, express in the physical. The subtle first - and then the physical. It could take years, or minutes. (Ever scared yourself sick or received some bad news and shortly thereafter felt physically ill? I know I have!)

The Problem

Our current Western Medical system is rooted in Biology and is fundamentally analytical, linear, and reductive in nature. Its' focus is primarily on the structure and function of the physical body alone.

My years of extensive experience working with Biofield Healing Immersion,® clearing belief systems, emotional release techniques, meditation, quantum physics, art, dance, ancient Yogic teachings, metaphysics, mysticism, visualization, numerous methods of spiritual healing and energy healing techniques, color therapy, sound healing, and more, have all lead me to the same conclusion:

We live in a vibrational universe....a huge ocean-like field comprised of vibrating particles of energy, light, and information.

Your emotional and physical pain - any symptoms that are bothering you - are trying to get your attention. They're trying to tell you that your life is off balance. Your energy field is disturbed and out of alignment with your true nature and what is best for you.

You are constantly sending out vibrational signals and in very simplistic terms, all health is a high vibration and all illness is a low vibration. Like vibration draws like vibration right back to itself. So if you are ill, unhappy, focused on "what's wrong" or on your dis-ease in any way, you are literally sending out a vibrational "call", a signal for MORE of the same to return to you.

Now I'm *sure* that is not what you want, right?

Reciting affirmations day and night will not solve this.
Positive thinking will not correct this.
You must learn to release and then access a higher vibration.

Your body is an amazing biofeedback feedback machine, and it's a metaphor for what is going on with you at a deeper level.

In today's world, it's so common for humans to be disconnected and out of touch with their true feelings, the wisdom of their body, and with the inner GPS system that we all come "hard-wired" with - our intuition.

But the thing is ...

In order to heal, you must feel.

Until you become willing to listen to the messages your body is sending you, to sort out your untrue beliefs and examine your conditioning from childhood, and learn how to release the resulting emotional pain from your energy field, you will continue to suffer and feel stuck or blocked in some way. You most likely will experience repeated painful patterns, no matter what you do to try and get rid of them.

EXERCISE
"Break Free From Painful Patterns"

<<<------------------->>>
INSTRUCTIONS For This EXERCISE:
Remember: find a safe place to complete the exercises. You should not be driving or operating any equipment or machinery, and it's best to do this sitting up rather than lying down. Some people may experience pressure in the head, slight dizziness, even nausea or other mildly uncomfortable symptoms as they complete these exercises, and even while reading through the book. If this happens to you, please know it's perfectly normal and indicates that you are receiving and responding to frequencies of healing. These are higher vibrations than you are used to and the discomfort normally passes quickly. Just breathe, relax, and allow them to integrate.
<<<------------------->>>

For this exercise, you'll need a pen and some paper.

The simple act of reflecting and recording your thoughts can and will start to bring up new awareness for you and to shift harmful, painful patterns...even patterns in your physical body.

As you complete this exercise, it's likely that pain will come up. Don't resist it. Remember, in order to heal, you must feel. Resisting feelings only keeps them stuck.

Below, you'll find a list of harmful behaviors that are the most common cause of pain and suffering. As you read each item, take a personal inventory. Write down what, if anything you do that relates to each item, and how it contributes to your pain, stress, and symptoms.

Then, ask yourself: What action steps will I take, beginning today, to reduce my pain, stress, and suffering?

Here's the list:

Ask yourself....Am I ?

- Resisting what is going on, being said, or happening?
- Not feeling my feelings?
- Being dishonest about my feelings?
- Taking things personally?
- Spending time with negative people?
- Gossiping?
- Not moving my body or exercising?
- Saying, "Yes," when I mean, "No"?
- Doing too much, or over-giving?
- Not doing enough, or holding back?
- Focusing on myself all the time?
- Focusing totally on others and forgetting to take care of myself?
- Taking on the problems of other people?
- Holding onto past people, places, and things I can't change?
- Not following my own inner guidance?
- Jumping to forgiveness when I don't truly feel it?

Note: This is only a partial list. What other harmful patterns come to mind? Jot them down now too.

Remember, this is a two-part exercise.

After you've identified your own behaviors and thought patterns that fall into this list, write down action steps you'll begin taking immediately to reduce your pain, stress, and suffering.

When you're ready, move on to the next chapter.

CHAPTER 3: The Doorways

We've talked about the energy-and-information field that surrounds you, and how *your body, your mind, and your emotions are the doorways to uncovering the hidden reasons you're not healing.*

Now it's time to learn more about each of these doorways.

We'll cover each type of doorway separately, and because one may resonate with you more than another, I recommend reading this entire chapter very carefully!

The information in this book truly only scratches the surface of what I have to share with you.. If you are ready to discover why thousands of my past clients have reported the complete and total elimination of their Chronic Pain, Depression, Anxiety, Chronic Fatigue, Trauma, Binge Eating, BurnOut, and much more...

If you are ready to receive my personal help and to experience for yourself my proven method backed by science known as Biofield Healing Immersion® ...

Then please accept my help and BEGIN RIGHT NOW to experience this incredible method for yourself. www.BiofieldHealingInstitute.com/dohps

The Physical Doorway

Some people perceive their pain most strongly in their bodies. I affectionately refer to these people as "the physicals." They receive feedback physically. They feel it in their bodies and are often the people who manifest things like headaches, earaches, pain in the neck, back, shoulders, and hips, and other physical pain.

I have found "the physicals" often receive diagnoses such as fibromyalgia, arthritis, inflammation, spinal disorders, and bone and joint conditions. They may suffer from things like TMJ, Carpel Tunnel syndrome, eye conditions, and frozen shoulders.

Often the pain seems to "move around" and may clear up in one area but then appear in a different part of the body. There is sometimes unpredictability and confusion about the pain and symptoms, as they "mysteriously" appear and disappear, changing from one area or symptom to another.

The Emotional Doorway

Other people receive feedback emotionally. They are "the feelers," and are often labeled "moody" and "too sensitive." They may be prone to feeling depressed, hopeless, anxious, sad, guilty, overwhelmed, confused, frustrated, fearful, angry, moody, spacey, and more.

Often these people are told "It's all in your head," or, "Don't be so sensitive," or, "There's nothing wrong with you," or, "You take things too personally," or, "You're so serious," or, "Can't you just let it go"?

I have found that "the feelers" often have trouble sleeping and suffer from mild to severe, and even chronic, insomnia.

It's very common for this group to have digestive disorders of all types including IBS, GERD, acid reflux, Colitis, Crohn's, and ulcers. Many of them complain of stomachaches, dizziness, nausea, vomiting, food intolerances, and all types of gastrointestinal issues.

These emotional processors often suffer from heart conditions, panic attacks, depression, immune disorders, cancers (particularly breast cancer), neuropathy, tingling and/or numbness of all types, and more.

The Mental Doorway

Still other people perceive their distress mentally. I call them "the thinkers." They're the ones who tell me, "I can't get a moment's peace. My mind races. It never stops. I'm always thinking. My head keeps me awake all night long."

They are the worriers tossing and turning at 2 a.m., trying to figure out what they should do.

"The " thinkers" constantly try to analyze and figure out what's wrong. They want to *know*. They research. They believe that if they just had the information, if they could just understand what's going on, they could find peace.

They think about their situation all the time, reviewing the problem, the circumstances, and possible solutions, over and over again, but never finding a way out. They often tell me they feel stuck or blocked no matter what they try.

"The thinkers" often try different methods to shut off their minds, such as keeping super-busy in order to distract themselves, focusing on other people's problems, drinking alcohol, taking drugs, smoking marijuana, shopping or spending money, having excessive sex, gambling, watching hours and hours of TV, and much more.

The Mind: Where It All Begins

Each of these avenues for perceiving dis-ease - physical, emotional, and mental - is connected to the other two, whether you realize it or not.

You may not be conscious of it, but you cannot have a physical pain without an emotion, or a thought, or both. Thoughts typically precede emotions, and emotions generate more thoughts. This is often a vicious, never-ending and Unconscious process.

When it comes to symptoms like anxiety, depression, and physical pain, the mind is often the real culprit.

"The thinkers" constantly give things, people, events, and situations *meaning*. They often make interpretations and assumptions subconsciously without checking out whether they're really true.

Here's the thing: *nothing means anything, except for the meaning you give it.*

The meaning you give an event or another person's behavior is learned and typically rooted in events that transpired from your past and usually dates back to your childhood.

As a child, through the age of approximately 8 years old, your brain is like a computer's hard drive. It doesn't have the ability to discern between what's true and what's false, or what's healthy and what will harm you. As a child, you simply take in everything that you see, hear, and feel going on around you. This forms the foundation for what you believe to be "the truth" and how life works.

The reticular activating system is a part of your brain that filters out everything that doesn't resonate with the "truth" your consciousness built upon that initial foundation. So unless you've ever started to look at your "truths" and question whether they were, in fact, true, then every situation you experience (even many, many years later) is infused with the meaning you assigned it early in life. There may be evidence of other "truths" right in front of you, but you won't even notice them.

Most people never examine their belief systems at all unless some kind of pain or suffering or unexpected (and usually unpleasant) pattern begins to repeat, and as a result, the person starts seeking answers.

For example, imagine growing up in a household where your father was abusive, maybe even physically violent toward your mother or you or your siblings. Imagine never knowing when he would be home, or what kind of mood he'd be in when he *was* home… maybe sometimes he could be really fun and charming, and then, seemingly out of nowhere, he could become mean, angry, even violent … and you never know why or what would set him off.

If there was screaming and yelling and lots of chaos around you like this, you may have made a decision very early in life that men are not safe, that they can't be trusted, that they always hurt you, they aren't there for you … or maybe you believe you and your needs don't matter, or that if you speak up and disagree, you'll get hurt.

Now this decision wouldn't likely be a *conscious* decision on your part. Rather, it would be an *unconscious* decision based on your environment. It would help you survive in the best way you knew how, yet it also would color your entire future without you realizing it.

Fast-forward 20, 30, 40, even 50 years. You find yourself in relationships with men who aren't there for you, or where there is abuse of some kind, including unpredictability and volatility similar to that with which you grew up. You can't seem to break this pattern, or you don't know how to get out, or you feel afraid to leave. Or, even worse, you hide it. You never talk about and instead keep it inside, as you try to figure out how you can fix it.

Perhaps somewhere along the line you would develop symptoms such as chest pains, stomach problems, or migraine headaches, but despite exams, testing, and more testing, the doctors can't find anything wrong with you.

Perhaps you experience joint pain, inflammation, numbness, panic attacks, depression, and anxiety. Maybe you are forgetful, have "accidents," have trouble concentrating or remembering things, or are told you have ADHD. Your doctors prescribe various medications but they don't seem to alleviate your symptoms.

This - or a similar situation - is a huge indicator that your pain and symptoms are *not* just physical. They are rooted in the underlying belief patterns and emotional reactions you developed earlier in life -as early as during your childhood but they are being "triggered" by something or someone in present time.

I call these original belief patterns, "home."

Right now, you may not even recognize how your current situation resembles "home." You might not be able to see that alternative choices exist. Why? Because the human psyche is programmed to go back "home" where it's familiar. Your beliefs therefore constantly come true, and show up in your world.

At some point, you may begin to see your pattern, and even to recognize that it resembles your childhood. You may start seeking answers or decide you absolutely will make different choices, but the pattern keeps repeating itself no matter what you do.

You may recite affirmations, create vision boards, go back and analyze your past until you are blue in the face, but nothing shifts, nothing changes.

This is an indicator that the belief system is still operating, and additionally, that you haven't learned to release certain **trapped feelings** from your childhood. The result: there is an **inner conflict** between two opposing parts of yourself.

Now, let's talk about your thinking. As I mentioned earlier, you have between 50,000 and 60,000 thoughts each day. Let that sink in for a minute. (Seriously – that is a *lot* of thought!)

Here's where it gets even more interesting: most of those thoughts are the same thought *in a different form.*

You have only about 10 unique thoughts each day, and you're thinking each one of them thousands of times.

That's how patterns are created. Your brain lays down neural networks, based on repetition. These patterns are colored by the "truth" you formed as a child.

It's a vicious cycle … until you learn how to release the patterns.

Emotions often manifest *after* your thoughts, and they wind up getting stuck and unexpressed. You may not realize the connection between these emotions and the thoughts that preceded them.

For example, one day, your boss seems upset about something. He has an angry look on his face; he seems tense, and maybe he even raises his voice. You don't know why, but all of a sudden you feel sick. You notice discomfort in your stomach, or part of your body begins to hurt. You get a headache, or begin to have pains in your chest.

You may notice *only* your physical aches and pains and dis-ease, not initially recognizing that underneath these aches and pains lies fear… triggered and ignited by a look, a tone of voice, or certain words or behavior that resemble "home": someone or something from your past.

It may happen in a nanosecond without you ever realizing that the belief, "Men will hurt me," is at the root. This was the original imprint, the original "decision," the original thought that caused an emotional reaction and now shows up disguised as physical symptoms. Your body goes into protection mode and sometimes the only way it knows to protect you is to make you "sick." Of course, this is just one example of how a thought can manifest as a physical symptom.

The Energetic or Spiritual Doorway

What the leading-edge Biofield Science is showing us is that around every living thing there is a field of energy and information, and that everything that has ever happened to us has been, and is being recorded in our field. It's like a vibrational library that houses all the information from our past. This is exciting news since scientific research has proven that energy is changeable! This means we can access this information, and that these patterns no matter how dysfunctional they may seem, or how long they've been there, have the potential to change.

I experience this constantly in my work with individuals and groups. Now I am able to access and work at the level of the quantum field, rather than only working at the mental or emotional level, which allows for the healing process to be rapidly accelerated.

I have developed the ability to immediately feel the disturbance patterns in the biofield, (whether I'm with you in person *or* remotely at a distance), and to then use the revolutionary Biofield Healing Immersion® method to shift this disturbed energy and information from a state of dis-ease, into the state of harmony and balance. Remember, your natural state *is* a state of harmony and balance.

Discover now and experience for yourself why thousands of my past clients have reported the complete and total elimination of their Chronic Pain, Depression, Anxiety, Chronic Fatigue, Trauma, Binge Eating, BurnOut, and much more…

Finally get UNstuck, UNblocked, and experience an extraordinary method of healing that has helped tens of thousands in over 150 countries to Live Pain Free…

Please accept my help and BEGIN RIGHT NOW to experience this incredible method for yourself. www.BiofieldHealingInstitute.com/dohps

EXERCISE
"How to Improve Your Health & Get More Of What You Want"

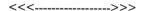

INSTRUCTIONS For This EXERCISE:
Remember: find a safe place to complete the exercises. You should not be driving or operating any equipment or machinery, and it's best to do this sitting up rather than lying down. Some people may experience pressure in the head, slight dizziness, even nausea or other mildly uncomfortable symptoms as they complete these exercises, and even while reading through the book. If this happens to you, please know it's perfectly normal and indicates that you are receiving and responding to frequencies of healing. These are higher vibrations than you are used to and the discomfort normally passes quickly. Just breathe, relax, and allow them to integrate.

<<<-------------------->>>

Take a moment to consider this as truth:

Your circumstances do not define your possibilities.

It's time to shift your perception.

What if **anything** *really* **were** *possible?*

Remember, your mind is often the root of where it all begins ... if you can change your thoughts, you can change your world, as you align with ultimate possibility.

Here's a technique for getting started:

At least once per day, write down something you already have or some evidence of something good in your life and the world.

For example, list one thing about your health that is working well, or one thing that you appreciate about yourself or someone else in your life.

Each day, find at least one new thing to add to the list.

Stay focused on what you **do** *have, on what* **is** *working in your health and your life. If you start to feel discouraged, come back to this list and remind yourself of what you already have to be grateful for. Remember, what you focus on increases! Focus on what you do have, not on what you do NOT have. You get more of what you focus on.*

When you're ready, move on to the next chapter.

CHAPTER 4: What Is Biofield Healing Immersion®?

Hopefully, since you've read this far, you now realize that your energy *is* your health.

Your energy shifts and changes all the time and is affected by numerous factors. The subtle level of energy shows up in your physical. Your thoughts and feelings (the subtle energy) determine your state of consciousness and your consciousness expresses as your physical body.

Now, it's time to become empowered.

No matter what your dis-ease, it *is* possible to increase your energy, and operate at a higher vibration, a higher state of consciousness. How? By releasing the low vibrational patterns of dis-ease, which are the root cause of your pain and suffering. Then you can return to your natural state of ease and comfort.

We call this a state of "coherency" in the biofield. It's a state of balance and harmony.

You see, Biofield Healing Immersion® is based on physics, rather than biology.

But before we go any further, I want you to be very clear on something: there is nothing you need to know or understand in order for Biofield Healing Immersion® to work.

In fact, "understanding" in its traditional sense—with your intellect—may actually get in the way of this healing modality.

The truth is, you may *never* fully understand this, or how it works. The greatest physicists in the country and the world are trying to explain it, to quantify it, both mathematically and theoretically.

I've been working in this field now for more than 30 years, and my understanding continues to shift and evolve.

So take this information in, but don't let yourself get caught up in struggling to truly understand the "how" behind the healing.

***

Biofield Healing Immersion® Bridges the Gap Between Science, Consciousness, and Spiritual Healing.

In simplistic energetic terms, I want you to think of your state of health as a very high energetic vibration, and the state of illness as a very low vibration ... an energetic vibrational pattern.

Now, here's where I might shake you up a bit (remember – open mind!): there is actually a state right now – at this very moment – a high vibrational state of consciousness where *you are not ill or in any pain.*

You just don't know how to access this state on your own. Everything going on with you - everything you call pain or dis-ease - is clouding *over* this harmonious, pain-free state of being. Most conventional healthcare practitioners, no matter how well meaning they are, aren't trained to help you access it. And as long as you are just focused on your body and on your symptoms, you won't find the solution.

But I can help you access that state, through Biofield Healing Immersion®.

Using The Biofield Healing Immersion® method, *I connect you to this higher-vibrational state where dis-ease does not exist* (and remember, this state already exists in the universe … it's the universe's natural, harmonious state.) I'm simply helping you access something you haven't been able to find or maintain on your own yet.

By bringing in coherent, harmonious higher vibrations, which communicate with the quantum field that surrounds your body, your entire being - physical, mental, emotional - begins to vibrate with a NEW pattern. The low vibration patterns (such as pain, depression, anxiety, etc.) cannot hold their form any longer and simply drop out of the field. They simply cease to exist.

Biofield Healing Immersion® is a non-linear process and works outside the realm of time and space. It is not a "thinking" process and doesn't require analyzing for it to work. It is not medicine in the conventional sense. It does not treat symptoms.

Instead, it addresses the *source* of your dis-ease energetically, the disturbed information patterns in your field, and works on all levels at the same time…the physical, mental, emotional, and spiritual.

As a result, your symptoms, even those you've had for years and years, may simply drop away, and you may experience immediate changes in the body, emotions, and the mind.

Again, you may not understand, intellectually, exactly *how* Biofield Healing Immersion® works, *but when you experience it, you know, deep in your bones, that something has happened.* You'll feel it or know it from within yourself.

"Something HUGE happened!! Something I feel in my bones and in my mind everyday. This truly was an amazing, life changing experience that is difficult to put into words. Whatever I write will not do my experience justice. During the sessions with Debora, I experienced healing beyond anything I had thought about or

dreamed about. Recurring issues/pain I'd been having for years with my low back were gone! Debora, you are a healing angel and I thank you so much!"
--Susie P., San Diego, CA

"I don't believe there are words to express the experience you have when healing is received. I came for one physical issue that had been harboring for months and months even with the assistance of herbs etc. Immediately I had relief, which was amazing and thrilling – the peacefulness came and physical issue was gone. As several days passed, I felt more at peace with myself and with who I was (this was a BIG THING also). I had some serious pain going on which I am sure related to things I have had for most of my life and incredible miracles happened with Debora… Sharing this is something that is so sacred and special it's difficult to describe other than I am totally blessed and thrilled to be on this fabulous journey knowing and experiencing what I have thus far. WOW!"
---Sonnie, Rancho Bernardo, CA

"As a scientist, bioenergy is not an easily approachable topic. To delve into the spiritual realm of healing, one needs a guide with uncommon ability to speak both science and spirit. For me, that guide is Debora. Her intelligence and ability to communicate logically as well as intuitively is a necessary bridge for me; not all healers have this. Debora is also an amazing teacher—she leaves no one behind. You'll leave with great inspiration and insight."
--- Neuroscientist, Ph.D Psychology

"I invited Debora Wayne to be a featured speaker at my event for holistic practitioners because I had experienced firsthand her healing energy and wanted to share it with my participants. Even with just a brief demonstration of Biofield Healing®, almost everyone in the room AND watching on the livestream was able to feel the healing effects that Debora transmits. Many people had actual healing results, even those at a distance not attending live. Some people felt very relaxed, their minds quieted down, and the typical overwhelm they feel melted away. They released anxiety, and for some, their pain disappeared, and they felt deep emotional release. One attendee who had a longstanding open wound that had not healed in months, saw it completely close up in just 24 hours after the healing session demo."
---Dr. Ritamarie Loscalzo, M.S, D.C, C.C.N, D.A.C.B.N Founder, Institute of Nutritional Endocrinology

"Working the Debora, I immediately felt relief from mental pain. My body was lighter and my mind clearer. Within 24 hours of my first Biofield Healing Immersion® session, I felt physical pain and emotional pain leave my body. My biggest discovery is that I can heal and control the problems that had kept me depressed, isolated, and blocked. I am a changed person. I find that opportunities and connection with others that I have always wanted are coming to me now without effort. Physically I am getting stronger and I love my life. Everything has changed in my life. I am excited about my future and so very grateful for the healing I have received."
---*Sharon H., Henderson, NV*

"I was a skeptic. I was also in a lot of pain and scared that I might face the rest of my life in pain. I was having severe joint, muscle, and neck pain. In the evenings it was hard to walk or sleep. My sessions with Debora, one by one, gave me back my hope, bliss, health, and opened my mind and heart in ways I will be forever grateful. I'm now pain-free. Don't live in pain. There is love, healing, and endless possibility through working with Debora."
–*Annette, La Mesa, CA*

You are a spiritual being - an energy being having a human experience.

Biofield Healing Immersion® has the potential to allow you to *experience* and connect to your multi-dimensional self.

Now to clarify, whenever I mention, "spiritual," I don't mean to imply something religious, "airy-fairy," or "woo woo."

I simply mean:

Everything is spirit ... you, me, all of life.

Spirit is energy and energy is spirit.

With Biofield Healing Immersion®, *your energy can and does change.* Everyone is different. You might experience small subtle changes like feeling more relaxed, or large dramatic "Hollywood Moments" that literally changes your entire life immediately. You may release your symptoms entirely, resolve inner conflicts and issues that have felt stuck, end the painful patterns in your relationships that you've been repeating for years, and your physical pain may finally stop.

As your vibration is elevated to a level where there is no dis-ease, you receive exactly what you need, and respond in your own unique individual, way.

Biofield Healing Immersion® is a process by which the old, outdated, learned patterns, (your conditioning), move out, and you return to your natural state which is whole, complete, and perfect … a state of ease, not dis-ease.

The beauty, and perhaps the best feature of Biofield Healing Immersion® is that it can and often does speed up the entire process of finding and releasing the *hidden* reasons, the *hidden* patterns and beliefs and triggers from your past that are causing the painful symptoms you're experiencing now. It may take you many years to uncover these on your own, or via some form of traditional "talk" therapy.

And the best part? It's often a very relaxing and enjoyable process where all you have to do is let it happen, while you observe the thoughts and feelings and sensations as they arise inside you.

You may find yourself, as so many of my clients do, feeling and acting quite differently, literally overnight! Issues and habits you've struggled with long-term simply wash away, without the need for willpower or discipline.

You may find that you are different, almost immediately. You feel changed.

You may find your voice. You may find yourself saying and doing things very uncharacteristic of the "old" you, without any effort on your part or without learning any new skills. You may easily begin to stand up for yourself, express your truth, stop worrying what other people think, feel free to speak your mind, follow your heart, and much more.

You may find your true calling, or the perfect job. You may see money and abundance of all types begin to flow. You may gain clarity on your life path, and find it easier to make decisions and healthy choices without mental strain or worry. Most people report feeling a deep sense of calm and inner peace and even a quiet mind, which they could never seem to achieve before. They begin to trust the process of life, and to feel happier and better about themselves, feel healthier and just all around more relaxed. Relationships often improve, and people report enjoying life a lot more.

It's truly nothing short of amazing!

If it sounds amazing to you too, and you'd like to get started and experience this for yourself right away, join me HERE: www.BiofieldHealingInstitute.com/dohps

The First Step to Healing

Remember: In Order to Heal You Must Learn to Feel.

You probably enjoy feelings such as happiness and joy, right? But what happens when you feel anger, guilt, fear or other "undesirable emotions"? Many people tend to shove certain feelings underground as if pretending to not have these feelings will make them go away. This never works, and in fact often leads to pain and other symptoms, sometimes slowly, sometimes quickly.

Remember feelings are not good, bad, right or wrong.
Just like there are no "bad" colors in the crayon box, there are no "bad" feelings.

The fastest way for healing to occur is first, to quit projecting fearful, negative "stories" about things that haven't happened yet into your future. Stop rehearsing these stories in your mind.

Next, stop resisting what is happening in your present and stop denying any feelings you have about this.

Do your best to feel your feelings fully. Observe what is happening in your current circumstances without interpretations. Often it's your interpretation of events that cause you to feel badly. Ask yourself if you are *certain* that your interpretation is 100% true. Most often it is not. The sooner you start to question your interpretations, and to *feel* your feelings, all of them, the faster they release and the faster you get to a state of peace.

All health originates from a state of inner peacefulness.

I realize that feeling feelings can be frightening to do on your own. It seems simple, sure, but it's not always easy.

To illustrate the powerful healing benefits of discovering and releasing *underlying hidden emotions*, I'd like to share with you an example from a former client and how she experienced complete recovery from a severe physical condition as a result of Biofield Healing Immersion®.

> Doctors told this 40 year-old woman who had been diagnosed with a brain tumor that she needed surgery, as well as a metal plate inserted into her skull, in order to have any chance of recovery. Her tumor had been pressing on a nerve that caused her to lose vision in one eye and consequently, she lost her driver's license as a result. You can imagine how this impacted every area of her life.

> This client refused the suggested medical treatment and somehow found her way into my office.

She agreed to complete a minimum of 4 Biofield Healing Immersion® sessions and during the second session she became aware of how extremely angry she was with certain intimate relationships as well as certain circumstances going on in her life. She now recognized that she had been allowing this to go on for quite some time and it was causing her a great deal of inner turmoil, as well as mental and emotional pain, and yet she had not done anything to try and remedy the situation. She had been keeping everything tucked away tightly inside, pretending it didn't exist.

Prior to our Biofield Healing Immersion® session she did not "see" any of this happening nor see her part in the situation.

During our healing session she began to "see" everything clearly. All the feelings she had been suppressing came up and began to release. The required actions that were needed in order to remedy the relationship challenges and other issues became crystal clear to her, and she felt completely confident, motivated, and ready to carry out these new actions immediately.

It's important to note that her clarity, awareness, and action plan was not the result of any discussion, analysis, or strategizing between the two of us.

Everything was revealed to this client directly from within herself, from within her own inner guidance system and occurred in complete silence during this session of Biofield Healing Immersion®,

She simply *knew* what to do. She saw her part clearly, stepped out of the role of "victim," and literally shifted "instantly" into feeling and behaving like an empowered woman.

As a result, within approximately one month, using no other form of therapy or treatment of any kind other than Biofield Healing Immersion®, this client's vision returned to 20/20, she was given back her license and the right to operate a motor vehicle, she became much happier, and continued to make healthier choices in all areas of her life. She even found herself finally improving her diet and nutrition, (which we never discussed at all) and which was something she had struggled with in the past.

Healthier choices just happened effortlessly now, and the most exciting news was that she was pronounced "tumor free" and was able to avoid surgery completely.

I've worked with SO many people suffering from a wide variety of symptoms, pain, and dis-ease of all types, and most of them are now living healthy, full lives. Nothing makes me happier or is more thrilling to me than to witness these recoveries!

Again, if you'd like to discover why and how Biofield Healing Immersion® may be able to help you identify and release your hidden reasons, help you to remove the root causes of your pain symptoms, so you can transform your energy and life...Please join me here for a deep, potentially life-changing experience: Contact@BiofieldHealingInstitute.com

Now, are you ready for an exercise?

EXERCISE
"Scanning"- A Powerful Tool for Clearing Dis-ease

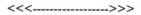

INSTRUCTIONS For This EXERCISE:
Remember: find a safe place to complete the exercises. You should not be driving or operating any equipment or machinery. Some people may experience pressure in the head, slight dizziness, even nausea or other mildly uncomfortable symptoms as they complete these exercises, and even while reading through the book. . If this happens to you, please know it's perfectly normal and indicates that you are receiving and responding to frequencies of healing. These are higher vibrations than you are used to and the discomfort normally passes quickly. Just breathe, relax, and allow them to integrate.

This exercise is best done sitting up, not lying down. It's more effective if you complete it while your eyes are closed, so read through the instructions, then take a moment to focus and close your eyes.

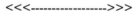

Let's Begin:

Take all your attention inside yourself.

Scan your body, from the top of your head to the tips of your toes, while you think about a situation in which you feel stuck or blocked or hurt.

You may instantly feel where there is pain in your body. If there is pain (or tension, stress, constriction, or tightness) in more than one place, scan your body and notice which pain stands out the most and begin there. Take your attention right to that area.

Notice the feelings that come up when you're thinking about this particular situation.

Imagine a little doorway in that part of your body, and open it up. Look inside and explore what's going on in there. What does it look like? What does it sound like? What does it feel like?

Explore the images, colors, thoughts, words, sounds, memories, everything you experience as you explore this area where you notice pain and/or discomfort of any kind.

Allow the feelings to come up. Speak to the feelings. Speak to the part of your body that's hurting, as if it's a person. Tell it that you're aware of it, and let it know you're not going to ignore it any longer.

Ask all the thoughts and feelings and images to come up, now, so you can experience them and feel them. Notice, listen, and observe, without applying any labels of good, bad, right, or wrong.

Trust the answers you get. Allow everything to come up.

Next, imagine that the pain, feelings, and symptoms in this area are now easily leaving your body, through that doorway, like smoke.

Allow it to drift away. Picture this or imagine it in any way you can.

You can use this process again and again to clear dis-ease from different parts of your body.

CHAPTER 5: Creating Change

Neuroscience has proven that there is a 4-step process to creating lasting change.

Part 1. Learn New Knowledge

You're learning new knowledge right now, aren't you? You've read this book, and you've discovered a new possibility exists. You now know that everything is energy, and all energy is changeable. You know that you have the ability to affect the energy that surrounds and flows through you, and that your body is designed for healing - it's designed to operate at a higher, healthier frequency. Remember, all mental, emotional, or physical pain is just a pattern, a vibration that is changeable!

Part 2. Receive Hands-On Instruction

The exercises you're using in this book are simple, yet extremely powerful. However, this is just the tip of the iceberg when it comes to all that I have to share with you.

There is a deeper, an actual ***experience*** of the Biofield Healing Immersion® method that goes beyond anything I could write or teach you. It goes *beyond* intellectual learning.

Join me here: **www.BiofieldHealingInstitute.com/dohps** and experience Biofield Healing Immersion ® yourself.

Part 3. Pay Attention

Notice what's happening. Notice when you're starting to slip into old mental and/or emotional patterns that don't serve you. The simple act of noticing when you do this begins to shift everything! If you can notice, and then become *willing* to drop the untrue thought that leads to painful emotions (drop the thought like it's hot!), then you can immediately begin to shift your pattern. If you're getting something positive out of the mental or emotional pattern or thought, then ask yourself what, specifically, you're getting out of it. But if it's about to take you down a dark and familiar path, be willing to drop it immediately and move forward. The key here is first to notice your thoughts and how they create your emotions and be *willing* to drop the thoughts.

Part 4. Repeat

Repetition is the key for your brain to lay down new neural patterns and create the synaptic connections that take place in your brain.

Once you get this process in place, through *repetition*, you'll eventually feel like autopilot takes over and the changes you wish to see will appear in your life. The effect will be cumulative over time.

You'll also begin to more quickly and easily notice when and where you are taking a certain thought, emotion, and/or experience and storing it in your body.

You'll have more choice over how you react to each experience. Pretty amazing, isn't it?

Life doesn't "just happen." It's all about choices. You have many more choices, and much more power, than you most likely realize, and your future is created by the choices you make today!

EXERCISE
"The Screen Door Technique - Rapid Release For Emotional Pain"

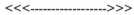

INSTRUCTIONS For This EXERCISE:
Remember: find a safe place to complete the exercises. You should not be driving or operating any equipment or machinery, and it's best to do this sitting up rather than lying down. Some people may experience pressure in the head, slight dizziness, even nausea or other mildly uncomfortable symptoms as they complete these exercises, and even while reading through the book. . If this happens to you, please know it's perfectly normal and indicates that you are receiving and responding to frequencies of healing. These are higher vibrations than you are used to and the discomfort normally passes quickly. Just breathe, relax, and allow them to integrate.

<<<--------------------->>>

It's time to begin creating change! You now know that physics shows us that everything is energy. You know that many of your mental and physical symptoms can be attributed to "stuck" energy patterns, and that these patterns can shift and change so they are vibrating at a higher, completely pain-free frequency.

You also know that in order to see these patterns, you must pay attention to them, not try to fight them, deny them, or avoid them!
Once you've begun to notice and pay attention to the patterns that are causing you emotional and physical pain, complete this exercise.

Imagine that your body, from the top of your head to the bottoms of your feet, is a screen door. A grid, with openings.

Feelings – of ANY kind - can easily pass through this screen door.

Instead of coming up against your solid body, or getting stuck in your body, these feelings can just pass right through. If it helps you to imagine these feelings as colored smoke, visualize them moving through the screen door that is your body.

Notice the feelings, feel them, but allow them to pass *through* that screen door.

They're not a part of you, they move *through* you.

This simple visualization exercise can provide a great beginning to healing, and can prevent further feelings or energy from getting "stuck" in your body and appearing as pain.

CONCLUSION

If you have ever asked yourself: "Why do I still hurt?" remember, there is *always* a reason.

The way to live pain-free is *not* to fight, resist, deny, suppress, or repress pain, emotions, or dis-ease of any type. The key that unlocks the door is to discover what it's trying to teach you.

Pain is always a gift.

Ask instead – What Can I Learn From This Experience?

Whether you are new to this type of understanding, or you have been working on yourself and exploring this subject for years, always remember to:

Be gentle with yourself

Be kind to yourself

Be patient with yourself

As you learn new ways of thinking and feeling

Treat yourself as you would

a small child entrusted to your care,

or someone you really, really love.

Keep in mind that you're seeking progress, not perfection, and that you should be gentle and kind with yourself as you're discovering and practicing new ways of thinking.

In our society, the idea that growth is some big, extroverted, dramatic, grandiose happening is a popular one.

The truth, though, is that although growth *can* be sudden and dramatic, often it is small and quiet. Growth is happening constantly whether you realize it or not, one small step at a time, and it's sometimes very subtle and not linear. In general, people in our society don't value the quiet, slow, small steps, so often they don't slow down enough to listen inside where we are able to recognize that change *is* happening.

You are growing *all* the time.

All health, all healing, all high states of consciousness, start from a state of peace and calm.

A higher state of being means you are aware that you have thoughts, emotions, and a body, but also aware that you are **not** your thoughts, emotions, or simply a body. You are much more than your personality.

A higher state of consciousness means you are aware of your connection to a power greater than your personality, aware that you are literally part of nature, one with everyone and with all that is. You recognize that you are made of tiny particles of energy, light, information, and love, and that there is no greater force in the entire Universe.

QUESTION: What do you need to do to connect with this higher state?

ANSWER (here's the shocker):

NOTHING!

Just Be Present. *Be.* Be Present to What Is.

You *already are* connected.

You may not realize it yet, or you may not see it or feel it because there are clouds" covering over the real you. Therefore, you may need to do some deeper work to release the thoughts and feelings that stop you from experiencing the connection, but – again - the fact is, you *are* already connected.

The Biofield Healing Immersion® method and all the tools I've shared with you in this book guide you in setting the proper foundation and developing greater awareness of the interconnection between your body, mind, emotions, and spirit so you can release the "clouds" that are covering over your natural state of peaceful, joyful, healthy *BEING*.

Biofield Healing Immersion® and the other tools I will continue to share with you in my various programs are designed to lead you to a total transformation and help you get your entire life on the right track for *you,* so you become at ease, joyful, and energetic in every way.

With practice, you'll be able to access this blissful state of peace and calm more easily and for longer periods of time. In fact, it may become your new normal.

As you change, some fear may come up. Don't avoid it; it's totally normal. Old trauma may come up, too. Pain, anger, frustration and old, stored-up emotions that imprinted on your energy field during past experiences … they may come up.

Don't resist this. Don't fight it. Instead, *feel* it.

It is just energy moving. This "coming up" allows the emotions and old experiences to move *through* you (just like in the exercise I shared in Chapter 5) and actually resolve. This is what it means to "let go."

When you do, you will finally heal all of those old patterns lingering in your field that affect your health in ways you likely can't imagine.

Although I've used the word, "heal" throughout this book, the truth is there is really nothing to heal. Instead, as you allow the painful feelings, traumas, and patterns to move out, you return to your *natural* state ... the state of ease and wholeness.

Health and wholeness *is* your natural state. You are already perfect, whole, and complete and there is nothing you lack.

***

If you have shown up here with me, and if you're still reading, it's because you're ready to do this! Some part of you may be afraid, or filled with doubt and despair, but you would not be reading these pages if another, perhaps wiser, "higher" part of you was not totally ready to receive this information, and to finally get your life back on track.

All that is required now is your willingness to begin—and continue—to practice the tools I've offered you.

For me, this has been a long, incredible journey from the wood floor of ballet school to the wood floor of my walk-in closet where I literally "hit bottom". The journey thankfully didn't stop there, but continued gifting me with "divine moments", leading me out of "health hell", and unexpectedly connecting me to both deep inner space, and the far reaches of the cosmos.

I'd love to join *you* and assist you on *your* journey, and save you years of time, money, and heartache as you attempt to dissolve your pain and patterns and return to the state of wholeness that is your birthright.

In Closing

> *"Take a chance! All of life is a chance. The person who goes the furthest is generally the one who is willing to do and dare."*
> *---Dale Carnegie*

I'd like you to consider something. All day long when the sun is shining, you cannot see the moon. It *seems* like the moon is gone. However, just because you cannot see it, doesn't mean the moon does not exist, or that it's gone or destroyed ... right?

You simply cannot **see** the moon at the present moment, even though you know it still exists.

With this in mind I'd like to ask you to read this message every single day:

"Hold the thought of total health, wholeness, happiness, even if these do not appear to be present in your current life."

Health is wholeness. Wholeness is health.

You were designed perfect, whole, and complete … lacking nothing.

You may not see the "proof" of your healing yet, but that doesn't mean it's not possible or true (remember, people once believed the earth was flat!).

Hold the thought of wholeness until you see it appear.

"Your imagination is your preview of life's coming attractions."
---Albert Einstein

Picture, see, and *feel* what it would feel like if you were *already* whole, perfectly healthy, happy, and living your ideal life. Sit quietly and imagine this so vividly that you can actually *feel* it as if it has already happened!

Repeat this practice daily and especially any time your mind wanders back to your old familiar story of woe, fear, and limitation…..and then, watch incredible changes begin to occur.

Stay focused on the possibilities rather than what seem to be your current limitations.

Practice the tools in this book again and again.

And whatever you do, *never give up.*
Taking New and Different *Action* is the Key.

I invite you next to discover and *experience* firsthand the power of Biofield Healing Immersion®, and to allow me to help you further. Let's add *your* story to the list of "healing miracles."

Join the thousands, from all over the world, who have benefited from this revolutionary method of healing. **www.BiofieldHealingInstitute.com/dohps**

As I mentioned before, the information in this book truly only scratches the surface of what I have to share with you and of what's possible for you as you begin a new journey to healing and optimum health.

If you want nothing more than to get your life back, to live more fulfilled, and experience more joy, and you're tired of feeling frustrated and disappointed, tired of trying to figure out what's wrong, and tired of trying "everything," only to continue experiencing the same old symptoms, then I invite you to try something new … something revolutionary.

Just go here to reserve your spot: **www.BiofieldHealingInstitute.com/dohps**

With Love,

Debora

"Ask and it will be given to you; search, and you will find; knock, and the door will be opened for you."

---Jesus

About Debora

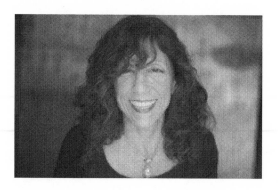

DEBORA WAYNE, founder of "The Pain Free Living Program®," is an internationally known pain release and energy expert specializing in helping those who suffer from Chronic Pain, Depression, Anxiety, Trauma, and more.

Her life-changing programs help people regain their energy, and get their lives back on track, while releasing the *hidden reasons* for pain and symptoms that don't and won't show up on medical tests.

Many of Debora's past clients have reported complete and total elimination of severe conditions even though nothing else they tried previously, worked. Since her own "health wake-up call" 31 years ago, Debora has been immersed both personally and professionally in the Healing Arts. Her life's work has evolved into an effective system that unites both science and spiritual healing, and is a unique blend of ancient techniques, modern discoveries from Physics and Neuro-Science, along with her own revolutionary method known as Biofield Healing Immersion®.

Debora has earned degrees and certifications in Psychology, Hypnotherapy, & Chemical Dependency Counseling, has 30 + years practicing and teaching the Art of Meditation, is a nationally recognized Fine Artist, a Certified Yoga Instructor, a Reiki Master, and Founder of The Biofield Healing Institute®.

FOR MORE INFORMATION regarding individual, group, online programs, & practitioner training:

Visit: **www.biofieldhealinginstitute.com** or Call 858-755-0883 NOW

Made in the USA
Middletown, DE
28 June 2019